7

secrets to Unlimited health:

Live long and live healthy

By

Thelma M. Smith

INTRODUCTION

Health is a state of being healthy physically, mentally and socially as well. It is not just the absence of disease,affliction, illnesses or infirmities. It is very crucial that one strives to live a healthy and long life.

Can we just be look at things objectively? Who would rather not get up each day with limitless health and imperativeness to start off their day with style?

All things being equal, It is really difficult to perform at top levels when you generally feel drained and debilitated. Everybody at some point have periodic cold or stomach upset at some point, however, Have you seen the best individuals appear to be almost strong each day,they appear to be invincible, Like they never appear to get worn out despite the fact that they have tons of work to oversee in their various organizations or even perform 7 hours straight in front of an audience.

It's unfathomable yet obvious, Effective individuals esteem themselves and health profoundly. That is, they put resources into their own health first and value their self more. They appreciate life, and don't need ailment or unhealthy thoughts to affect their direction in life.

To keep you at your best, the following are six (6) straightforward propensities that will assist you in being healthy physically, mentally and socially.

1.

Eat Right

Eating the right food sources and the perfect proportions of food varieties can and will assist you with living a longer, better and healthy life. Research shows that numerous diseases, for example, diabetes, coronary illness, and hypertension can be forestalled or constrained by just eating right. Getting the right supplements your body really needs is very important, for example, calcium and iron. Also monitoring your weight can help. Attempt to balance the calories you get from food with the calories you use or burn when you work. Keep in mind, you can start at anytime to eat right! It's not too late. In addition to that, it is critical to not skip breakfast, breakfast is very important to keep your body in check. Research shows that healthy breakfast helps balance the body metabolism and also help prevent poor nutrition. Skipping breakfast turns out to be more normal as kids progress in years. Some schools have presented breakfast programs since they were worried about kids who skip breakfast. Concentrating on shows that kids in different occasions perform better at school when they eat. They are likewise bound to keep a sound weight when they consume a sound breakfast.

Then again, grown-ups who have healthy breakfast are likewise more reasonable, be of sound weight and more useful at work. Breakfast is a approach to launch your digestion in the first part of the day ,It is a method for reminding your body that now is the right time to start up!

Nutritious breakfast is like an engineer of the body system.

You really want to get great sustenance from the calories you take? At all expense, stay away from "void" calories. So what does it mean? It essentially implies food or beverages with calories not comprised of fundamental macro nutrients Proteins,Carbs and Fats. An incredible illustration of void calories drink is liquor. They give no supplements to your body except for those undesirable calories that make you fat.

Discussing fat, additionally, keep away from food with loads of undesirable fats or added sugars or both. These will genuinely make you undesirably fat especially if consumed in enormous amounts and frequently.

Secrets to get in shape;

Select filling, low-calorie food as opposed to sweet, fat-rich calorie-thick food!

Here is a model, There are two food varieties on the table, One is a piece of carrot cake, and another is a pack of carrots. Both contain some similar measure of calories.

Knowing that if you eat a piece of carrot cake, you will not get full enough to help your wellbeing and most likely you even crave for more. In any case, suppose you

eat similar number of calories as carrots. All things considered, you get the calories in addition to an entire pack of extraordinary supplements and you'll feel very full. That's the logic.

Remember that most young ladies opt in to eat something like 120 or 160 void calories daily. How might you stay away from void calories? Have a go at cutting back on sweet soft drinks, natural product drinks, frozen yogurt, treats, and cake.

Here are a few supportive tips of practicing good eating habits

Eat different varieties of food, especially;

- Vegetables such as green leafy and deep yellow veggies
- Fruits such as Pick berries, melons, citrus natural products or juices.
- Whole grains, like oats, grain, corn, wheat, rice, oats.
- Whole grain breads and oats.
- Dry beans such as soybeans, naval force beans and red beans, peanuts, lentils and chickpeas.

Eat food low in fat, cholesterol and saturated fat, particularly:

Fish

Poultry arranged without skin, lean meat and Low-fat dairy items.

2.

Be Genuinely Active

According to research, bring active can assist with forestalling not less than six illnesses such as coronary illness, hypertension, stoutness i.e over weight, diabetes, osteoporosis, and mental problems like depression. Physically moving will help you feel improved and remain at a sound weight and mentally sound.

In addition to that, various examinations has found that exercise alleviates misery. Just moving your body can really take care of individuals in misery. Actual activities likewise block negative contemplations or divert individuals attention from day to day stresses. Some even call it a functioning type of reflection.

Furthermore, interacting with others gives a chance to expanded social contact. Increment wellness might lift your state of mind and even further develop rest pattern.

Research proposes that lively strolling around can be basically the same for you as an action like running. A decent rule of thumb to observe is to do a sum of thirty minutes of steady work or exercise, like quick strolling, most days of the week.

Before you begin being truly Active;

- Talk with your doctor or personal advisor about ways of getting everything rolling.

- Pick something that squeezes into your day to day routine, like strolling, cultivating, raking leaves, or in any event, cleaning windows as well.

- Pick an action you like, like walking, swimming, dancing, etc.

- Attempt another activity, such as trekking or hiking.

- Request that a companion start with you, or join a gathering.

Try not to stop,keep going, do not quit!

- Set aside a few minutes for active work, begin gradually, and keep at it.
- Assuming that the weather conditions is awful, attempt an activity show on television, watch an activity tape in your home, stroll in the shopping center, or work around the house.

Physical tasks Rule

Here is a phenomenal rule to keep;

- ⬚ Doing even the littlest is better than not doing at all; For example if you no active work,nothing at all to keep your body and soul active, begin by doing some, and bit by bit you develop your self.

- Stay Active always, ideally the entire is okay (Still make time to rest), days and consistently.

- Take record of your activeness each day

- Do muscle reinforcing exercises at least somewhere around two days every week.

3.

Keep a positive attitude at all times.

The attitude and mindset you maintain at all times is very crucial. Positive mindset is infectious, negative is as well. Individuals around you will pick your psychological temperaments and are affected as needs be one way or the other.

Going everyday with pessimistic mindset continually can gauge an individual down both physically, mentally, socially and intellectually. Moving these negative thoughts into positive ones is a significant contemplations. Negative thoughts can weigh down your day and negatively affect your own life. Many individuals don't remember to drive the considerations away and it is vital we do. However we can really control what considerations we choose to let influence us,when we become conscious of our own thoughts.

We should set aside a few minutes for good energy. It is a given that if you encircle yourself and your existence with pessimism, you will wind up in a terrible place. Make time in your day to always do things that satisfy,try as much to distract your self when ever negative energy sets in.

This can be a side interest,such as perusing, sports or exercise. Whatever can be zeroed in on and delighted in by you is a decent interruption from pessimism. If you are too centered around parts of your life that don't advance as it should, spice it up with positive reasoning, if not, those things will wind up controlling your life.

While rehearsing the strategy of overlooking negative considerations, you can likewise work on presenting energy in those conditions. Consider anything positive to supplant your negative contemplations. Rather than getting down about something or letting it take control of you, view it from the bright side of life,as something cheerful and utilize this hopeful remembrance of it to supplant your negative thoughts on it. Rehearsing this over the long run, your brain will start to zero in on the great as opposed to the terrible. Finding a decent way to offset your feelings is vital to being a cheerful and effective individual. Deal with your whole self by ensuring negative contemplations don't run your life for you. So your body will not be much affected.

These individual propensities will work on your general life and help you live more healthy.

The following are 6 hints to defeat negative considerations.

Positive Reasoning Made Simple;

1. Meditate

2. Do Yoga

3. Encircle yourself with positive individuals.

4. Recollect that nobody is great and push your self.

5. Remember Your Good fortune,and be grateful.

6.Try not to play the victim card. You make your life assume liability.

Subsequently,Always make sure to keep an inspirational perspective. It has an enormous influence on your general prosperity and health. Research has it that a number of health benefits associated with optimism and positive attitude, includes less depression, reduced risk of death from cardiovascular problems,reduced anxiety disorder and prolonged health. Always remember attitude is everything!

4.

Depend on experts

Yes,trusting an expert,a professional, a specialist is a way to go. There are different sorts of disease known, and each type requires its own specific treatment. Early finding and quick diagnosis will permit these medicines to start rapidly in supposed manner, allowing the patient the most elevated opportunity for an effective recuperation.

According to research,nearly 1.5 million people are diagnosed with some form of cancer lin the United States, and cancer kills over 500,000 people annually in the United States alone, If calculated worldwide that number is closer to 12.5 million cases diagnosed and perhaps over 7million deaths from cancer. Thirty to forty percent of these cases could be prevented and close to one third cured if detected and diagnosed early enough. Depending on professionals will help you as an individual prevent and detect any disease that could pose a threat to your life.

So the inquiry you need to pose to yourself is, are you able to accept you are healthy in light of the fact that you feel fine or how about it be more savvy to make an arrangement with a specialist you are comfortable with, particularly on the off chance that it has been more than a year since you have been checked, and go get a test. What do you have to lose? A couple bucks for the visit? Could you at any point put a cost on your wellbeing? Or then again considerably more, might you at any point put a cost on life?

One ought to get yearly actual examination to ensure everything is as it ought to be. There is no mischief getting standard check ups as it's great for your own body. Do bosom or testicular self-tests and get dubious moles looked at. Getting tests consistently will help you out alot, supposing and when something is unusual in your body, you will get to be aware of it at the ideal time and hence your doctor will make appropriate recommendations for early treatment.

Additionally, you should assume a functioning part to benefit from your specialist's visit. That is to capitalize on your examination, here's a speedy agenda to consider;

- Survey your family health history,this will help you know if anyone in your family has a history of disease that might be hereditary example Alzheimer, cancer etc.
- See whether you are expected for any broad screenings or inoculations
- Record a rundown of issues and inquiries to take with you

During your real specialist's visit, don't be modest about getting your inquiries replied. Likewise, If your primary care physician opens up to you regarding about any unambiguous wellbeing issues, go ahead and notes. Time is in many cases restricted during these tests,So do as much to understand what is going on with you and what is expected. Since you came set and prepared with your notes and all, you're certain to take advantage of your test.

Standard tests and regular check ups will furnish specialists with a method for detecting any medical problems from the get-go. Exams consolidate a few tests, including safeguard screenings and actual assessments, to really take a look at patients' ongoing wellbeing and also If any issues of concern are found, your doctor will give you notice of treatment plans and ways that you can forestall medical problems later on.

Some Well known health checks include;

- Diabetes checks
- Pulse test
- Cervical smear tests for women
- Cholesterol level checks
- BMI and obesity tests

5.

Get Sufficient Rest

Rest misfortune and rest issues are among the most widely recognized triggers of ill-health. And it is every now and again neglected. The body needs rest to perform at its best, denying your body the rest it needs negatively affect wellbeing, giving the body adequate rest does not just help the body perform at it's peak, in addition it is likewise expected to take a toll on health. Effective individuals plan time to rest.A person who is competent must find time in his/her busy schedule to rest. Resting is as vital to your wellbeing just as eating appropriately and working out. It is really harming to your wellbeing to really work just hard without getting enough rest. However, many individuals are doing this consistently. In America, everything is done in a hurry and at a rushed speed. Yeah it is good to hurry but it is compulsory to rest!!! Take a break,No one will sue you.

According to Research ,It is assessed that 50-70 million US grown-ups have rest problem.

Prominently, wheezing and snoring is a significant mark of obstructive rest apnea.

Absence of rest can influence your general wellbeing and make you inclined to serious ailments.

Which may incorporate;

- Diabetes
- Heftiness
- Hypertension
- Coronary illness

Here's a question to answer;

What amount of Rest does our Body need? And how much of it would we say we are Getting?

Just as Evey individual is different,So it is for our body balance and the work we do. How much rest we need at any point is different amongst people, yet by and large it changes as we grow older. That is to say that,the amount of rest persons aged 60 years and above needs will be different from the one someone younger will need.

Well on an Average,it is expected to rest for at least 9-10 hours each day,to keep your health in check.

Tips for Hygienic Rest

- The advancement of good rest propensities and standard rest is known as rest cleanliness. The following accompanying rest cleanliness tips can be utilized to further develop rest.
- Set a time to Head to sleep simultaneously every night and wake simultaneously each morning.
- Keep away from enormous feasts before sleep time
- Keep away from nicotine

- Keep away from caffeine and liquor near sleep time

The following are five manners by which a decent night's rest can help your wellbeing;

1. Rest supports your mental health

2. Rest forestalls diabetes

3. Rest can keep you fit.

4. Work averts coronary illness

5. Rest boost immune system.

6.

Maintain good Relations

One need to be socially healthy and having a good relationship with people will accelerate your social health. Don't just be nice,be kind to people.Render help when and which ever way you can. People will have many good things to say about you and this will as well put a smile on you face.

A person who is able to feel other's pain is considered human.

n the office where you work,go out for dinner nights with your colleague(s), you can as well eat lunch together.This will help you get to understand each and every one of them better. Be an advocate for peace and watch good people being drawn to you by a force that shines within the goodness in your heart.

Live your life to the fullest,and you will be thankful you did!

6.

Don't let your life be all about work (Take time off work and go on vacation)

Don't let your life be all about work!! Make time for your self to breath. Although numerous Americans get paid time off work, and 96 percent of individuals perceive its significance, Just 41% of workers plan to fully utilize all of their vacation days. Getting much needed rest helps us relieve distress and that has long run good wellbeing suggestions. People who just took one vacation at maybe seven years intervals or less were almost multiple times bound to experience a cardiovascular failure or foster coronary illness than the people who took time out at any rate to get-away from work consistently, The New York Times reports.

Everybody needs a get-away time sometimes,as it has significant impact on our health and life. Obviously, stress is definitely not something to be thankful for. Indeed, even individuals who guarantee to adore the high-forced way of life will concede, in their calmer minutes, that there are times when they simply need to move away from everything, if by some stroke of good luck for a brief time frame.

Vacations can possibly break into the stress cycle. We rise out of a fruitful get-away inclination prepared to take on the world once more. We gain viewpoint on our concerns, get to unwind with our families and companions, and get a break from our typical schedules.

Meeting individuals from different societies will instruct you that how you've been taking a gander at the world isn't the way every other person does. Your point of view could have a few significant vulnerable sides, truth be told. Seeing the world for yourself will work on your vision and your grasp on the real world.

In addition to that, Assuming you're between occupations, schools, children, or connections, around

the world travel can be an ideal method for moving from one of these life stages into your next incredible experience. A major vacation won't simply slide your progress into the following phase of your life, it'll allow you an opportunity to consider where you've been, where you're going, and where you need to wind up.

Seeing the world gives training that is totally unimaginable. Travel shows you economy, legislative issues, history, topography, and social science in an exciting and active way that no class will. It causes you to feel invigorated.

We're constantly informed that to look for satisfaction, you want to attempt to live in the second. Furthermore, it feels remarkably difficult to do this during the time spent your everyday work and amidst schedule. You've seen everything previously, so your mind moves in a routine movement simply cruising everything by. However, when you travel, your psyche is there, you experience such a great amount interestingly without any work, and you're available at the time. It's no big surprise so many

individuals become dependent on voyaging. It's a steady surge of adrenaline and experience.

The ideal method for revitalizing yourself, and can be an incredible method for stirring up your life

In conclusion

Health is wealth! Take care if your health. Don't slave away and die in silence. At some point in your work life,give your self a break. No one brags with the suffering and stress life brings.

Be responsible for you, say where it hurts and get it fixed!

Give your body what it needs and your health will appreciate you!